医学・生命科学書
英文出版のすすめ
―著作を志す人へのメッセージ―

Publishing Medical and Scientific Books in English:
A Message to Prospective Authors

大垣　雅昭

メディカル・サイエンス・インターナショナル

Publishing Medical and Scientific Books in English:
A Message to Prospective Authors
First Edition
by Mark Ohgaki

© 2019 by Medical Sciences International, Ltd., Tokyo
All rights reserved.
ISBN 978-4-8157-0150-5

Printed and Bound in Japan

献　　辞

To the memories of

Christian C. Febiger Spahr

and

Joseph W. Lippincott, Jr.,

who taught me the business of publishing and selling medical books.

出版用語の使用について

1. 本書で使用する出版用語は，海外出版社との交渉時に役立つよう，日本語と英語を併記した。
2. 次の用語は英語のままで使用した。

Acquisition Editor(s)

　書籍出版のために，企画を取得し，審査し，契約する権限をもつエディターの呼称。経験豊富な編集者が選ばれ，出版社により異なる役職名(5.4 参照)が使われている。

Prospective Author(s)

　将来，本の著者になってもらえそうな医師や研究者のこと。

Quality book(s)

　良質で類書と区別のつく個性的なアイデアや創意に基づく本。常時出版していると Quality publisher と認められるようになる。

目　次

はじめに　　　　　　　　　　　　　　　　　　　　　　　　　　　　*viii*

第1章　出版社の使命　　　　　　　　　　　　　　　　　　　*1*

1.1　Are you a Prospective Author ?　　　　　　　　　　　　　*2*

1.2　医学・生命科学書の種類　　　　　　　　　　　　　　　　*3*

第2章　計画と準備　　　　　　　　　　　　　　　　　　　　*5*

2.1　Quality book を目指す　　　　　　　　　　　　　　　　　*6*

2.2　Quality book のキーワード　　　　　　　　　　　　　　　*6*

　2.2.1　着　想　　　　　　　　　　　　　　　　　　　　　　*6*

　2.2.2　ニーズ　　　　　　　　　　　　　　　　　　　　　　*7*

　2.2.3　読者層　　　　　　　　　　　　　　　　　　　　　　*7*

　2.2.4　コミュニケーション　　　　　　　　　　　　　　　　*7*

2.3　執筆の動機と構想　　　　　　　　　　　　　　　　　　　*8*

　2.3.1　動　機　　　　　　　　　　　　　　　　　　　　　　*8*

　2.3.2　判　型　　　　　　　　　　　　　　　　　　　　　　*8*

　2.3.3　単独・共同執筆　　　　　　　　　　　　　　　　　　*9*

　2.3.4　編集・監修書　　　　　　　　　　　　　　　　　　　*9*

第3章 執筆の要点と問題点 — 11

3.1	文　体 — 12
3.2	パラグラフ — 12
3.3	スペリング，略語，用語 — 12
3.4	人称，時制，動詞の態 — 13
3.5	明快で正確に — 13
3.6	動　詞 — 14
3.7	慣用句 — 15
3.8	副　詞 — 16
3.9	接続詞 — 16
3.10	代名詞 — 16
3.11	現在分詞と不定詞 — 17
3.12	批判と引用 — 17
3.13	著作権の取り扱い方 — 18
3.14	用語の調べ方 — 18

第4章 出版社を選ぶ — 21

4.1	図書館と書店を活用する — 22
4.2	研究仲間や同僚に訊く — 22
4.3	学会展示場で出版社に接触する — 23

第5章 企画書の作成と審査 — 25

5.1	企画の「狙い」，「目的」と「範囲」 — 28
	例文1：基礎免疫学 — 29

目　次

例文2：病理学総論 ……………………………………… 30

例文3：標準外科手術法 ………………………………… 31

例文4：小児の複雑な足奇形 …………………………… 33

例文5：不整脈 …………………………………………… 35

例文6：頻　拍 …………………………………………… 37

例文7：関節液分析 ……………………………………… 38

5.2　読者層・マーケット ……………………………………… 39

5.3　競合書 ……………………………………………………… 39

5.4　企画書の送付先 …………………………………………… 41

5.5　企画の審査 ………………………………………………… 42

第6章　契約締結→そして出版へ …………………………… 45

6.1　契約書 ……………………………………………………… 46

6.2　著者の責務 ………………………………………………… 47

6.3　編集と制作 ………………………………………………… 48

付　録 ……………………………………………………………… 49

1.　許可申請の手紙（見本）…………………………………… 50

2.　語句の使用法 ……………………………………………… 51

3.　海外の医学・生命科学系出版社リスト ………………… 60

引用文献/参考文献 ………………………………………………… 64

あとがき …………………………………………………………… 65

著者プロフィール ………………………………………………… 66

vii

はじめに

　優れた研究者は優れた教育者であると言われている。研究と教育の特性を，医師や研究者がどうデザインしていくかという発想が重要だ。

　医学・生命科学分野で，海外の学術誌に研究論文を発表することと，ポスドク，レジデント，学生の研修や教育のために書籍を作り出す仕事とが両立できるのであれば，研究と教育の融合と言えるだろう。

　本書の目的と範囲は，医師や研究者が医学や生命科学分野で，本を英語で執筆し，海外の出版社に提案し，契約締結を経て，出版に至るまでのプロセスと約束ごとを簡潔に示すことである。

　著者が企画書に記述する"Aim, Purpose and Scope"は，出版社の acquisition editor が最初に読む情報なので，本の内容を適切に伝えるものでなければならない。英語が自国語の 7 人のドクター（氏名を伏す）が書いた「例文 1〜7」は本書のハイライトである。是非とも参考にしていただきたい。

　利用が普及している PDF やデジタル化した内容には触れず，極力これまで思索してきた著作の本質と英文執筆の原理 philosophy を示すようにした。

　英語で執筆し出版にこぎつけるまでには，膨大な時間と労力が必要だ。しかし，著者が知的チャレンジの結果として，完成本を手にしたときのよろこびは何物にも代え難い。

　日本人著者による専門書や教科書が世界の読者に向けて刊行されるために，この小冊子の内容が少しでも役立つのであれば望外のよろこびである。

2019 年 1 月

大垣　雅昭

第 **1** 章

出版社の使命

Medical knowledge is not the property of a single nation but the
most prized possession of the entire human race.

—— Eugene Braunwald, M. D.

（Harrison's Principles of Internal Medicine, 15th Edition 中国版の序文から引用）

Are you a Prospective Author ?

Information for Prospective Authors

If you are preparing a manuscript for publication, Lea & Febiger will welcome the opportunity to consider it.

Write to:

Martin C. Dallago
Executive Editor
Lea & Febiger
600 Washington Square
Philadelphia, Pa. 19106

　これは，フィラデルフィアの医学書出版社 Lea & Febiger（現在は合併により Lippincott Williams & Wilkins, Inc.）の部門別カタログに載っていた広告である。同社は，Gray's Anatomy, Joslin's Diabetes Mellitus, Merritt's Textbook of Neurology, Wintrobe: Clinical Hematology, Bonica: The Management of Pain などの名著をかつて出版したことで知られているが，新しい著作者を探している編集者の心構えを伝えるため冒頭に引用した。

　出版事業は，まず良質でニーズがある書籍を企画することから始まる。出版社は，どんな内容の書籍が求められているかを調査し，需要動向と変化を予測して，その企画実現に向けて最適な著者に執筆を依頼する。独創性のある企画は，研究や教育の現場での経験や着想から生まれることが多いので，出版社はこのような企画の開発に真剣に努力している。優れた企画と優れた著作者の開発こそが出版社の使命である。

第1章　出版社の使命

1.2　医学・生命科学書の種類

　執筆には綿密な計画と準備が必要だが，どんな種類の本を書くのかを最初に決めないと何も進展しない。書籍の種類と名称は，体裁，内容，表現形式などから次のように分けられる。

Textbook	テキストブック，教科書
Atlas	アトラス，図譜，図解書
Text-atlas	テキスト・アトラス（ミックス型）
Synopsis	シノプシス，要約書
Monograph	モノグラフ，研究論文集
Proceedings	プロシーディング，（学会などの）会議録

　また，1人で書くのか，共同執筆するのか，寄稿者の原稿を集めて責任編集・監修するのかなどにより，次のようにも分類できる。

Single-authored book	単独執筆書
Co-authored or Multi-authored book	共著，多著作者書
Edited or Co-edited work	編集，共同編集書

第 2 章

計画と準備

2.1 Quality book を目指す

出版社は，いつも質の良い本を出そうと努力している。質の悪い本は，どんなに宣伝しても，またどれほど販売に力をいれても売れない。出版社は Quality book を出版することにより，目標とする読者層 Target reader を確実に獲得することができ，著作者は独創的な内容と努力に対して正当な評価を受け，また著作は適切な間隔で改訂を行えば定本として存続する。

書店で医学・生命科学分野の洋書売場を眺めると，よくもこんなに多くの本が出版されているものだと驚く。2,000 ページを超える大型の内科学や外科学のテキストブックから，100 ページ前後のミニ・アトラスに至るまで多種多様な本が並べられている。だが，このような既刊書の単なる模倣執筆で成功を収めることは困難であり，海外の一流出版社は，パクリ本や安易に仕立てた原稿はアクセプトしないことを知っておくべきである。

2.2 Quality book のキーワード

The publication of a book begins with an idea and a need.
Karen Berger, Editor, C. V. Mosby, St. Louis[1]

2.2.1 着 想——*idea*

優れた本は新しいアイデアに基づく企画から生まれる。アイデアは研究や教育現場での閃（ひらめ）きや，ちょっとした思いつきから出てくることが多い。したがって，アイデアが浮かんだらすぐノートし，後

日いろいろな観点から調べてみるようにしたい。類書の有無，出版されていたらどんな内容か，著者は，出版年は，ページ数は，などをチェックしてみよう。類書があっても，自分のアイデアに新味があり，違いが出せるのかがポイントになる。

2.2.2　ニーズ —— *need*

著者は，本の生命である内容 contents を創造する人であるから，教育や専門分野についての十分な知識と，読者に対する鋭敏な感覚をもつことが必要である。コンテンツは教育上，または専門的にみて価値があるかどうか，読者のニーズに合致しているか，タイムリーか，類書と違った特色があるか，などの諸点を執筆中に絶えず自問しなければならない。最近のマーケティング戦略では，需要demand はクリエートするものだが，そこには顧客(読者)のニーズが存在することを前提としている。

2.2.3　読者層 —— *reader/market*

テキストブックを書くのか，モノグラフを書くのかより，当然ながら読者層が異なる。対象とする読者をどこに求めるかによって，着想の狙い aim，目的 purpose，および範囲 scope が具体化する。読者層の中心をどこにするかを明確にせず，多目的で広範な内容の本を書く人がいるが，焦点の定まらない本に良書はない。結局はどの読者層にもアピールせず不成功に終わってしまうことになる。

2.2.4　コミュニケーション —— *communication*

著者と出版社間の良好なコミュニケーションが quality book を生むと言われている。

特に編集部門のスタッフとの信頼関係で仕事が進行するので，良書を出版するという双方の熱意とグッド・コミュニケーションが不可欠である。

2.3　執筆の動機と構想

2.3.1　動　機 —— *motivation*

著作には，多大な時間と労力を消費するもので，著者本人の努力はもとより，同僚や家族の協力なしには到底完成するものではない。特に大型書を執筆するとなると，資料の収集・分類・整理から，原稿執筆（入力）・図表・アートワークの準備に至るまで，膨大な作業が待ち受けており，またかなりの金銭的出費を伴う。反面，執筆により高額の印税収入 royalty income を得られるケースは極めて稀で，したがって，単に金銭的な報酬に基づく動機で執筆すると失望する。しかしながら，執筆活動は人間の専有する知的挑戦のプロセスであり，完成した quality work は業績として正当な評価を受けることになる。

2.3.2　判　型 —— *format*

日本人医師や研究者が海外の出版社に初めてアプローチする場合は，コンパクトな本を提案すると受理され易い。米国では，サイズが 7×10 インチ（約 178×254 mm）の本が多いが，初めての著作者はこれより小型，例えば 6×9$\frac{1}{4}$ インチ（約 152×235 mm）で 200 印刷ページ位の本を企画すると手頃であろう。契約書で完全原稿 complete manuscript の提出期限が設定されるので，18 か月間位で仕上がる本を目標にすると現実的である。

2.3.3　単独・共同執筆

　原稿は手書きでも PC 入力でも，最初から英語にすべきである。最終原稿は，英語が母国語のスペシャリスト——できれば，同じ専門分野で，海外の出版社から本を出版した経験があるエキスパート——に十分な時間の余裕をみて，英文の誤りを訂正したり，弱点を補強してもらい，最後に自分で内容を吟味して完全原稿に仕上げると万全である。企画の概要 outline を組み立てた段階で，このようなスペシャリストに共著者になってもらうのもよい方法である。

2.3.4　編集・監修書

　多数の寄稿者 contributors から原稿を集めて責任編集または監修する企画には，深い学識と豊富な経験が必要である。主題別にエキスパートを注意深く選ぶことが重要で，また当然のことながら，寄稿者によりアプローチの仕方に個人差が出たり，文体も異なるため，編集または監修者は原稿を企画の方針に沿って統一し，調整する能力をもたなければならない。

第3章

執筆の要点と問題点

> Medical authors must learn to write as educators learn to teach. You should learn to make your subject come alive: to make it meaningful, and to make it appeal to both the intellect and imagination of your readers.
>
> Anitra Peebles Sheen, Medical writer[2]

3.1 文 体

対象とする読者を常に念頭におき，文章のスタイルは，学生やレジデント向けか，広い意味でのスペシャリスト moderate specialists 向けにするのか，研究仲間のスペシャリスト向けに書くのか，一貫性があり読みやすい文章で書く。

3.2 パラグラフ

各パラグラフは単一の思考とその内容を記述するものなので，活字を詰め込むと読者は疲れる。各パラグラフは 125 語以下に保つようにし，それ以上になるようであれば分割を考える。

3.3 スペリング，略語，用語

英国式と米国式のスペリングをもつ語がある。同一語は全体を通じて同一のスペリングにする。番号，記号，略語は統一性をもたせる。特に略語は多用せず，各章の冒頭ページまたは初出の個所で意味を明確にしておく。実験室，検査室，また特定の病院や研究所だけで通じる用語は，すべて国際的に理解される用語に変える。

第3章　執筆の要点と問題点

3.4　人称，時制，動詞の態

　適切な人称 person，時制 tense，動詞の態 voice を使用する。著者が実践したことを述べるのには「I」か「we」を，指示するのには「you」か命令形を，また既に生じたことを書くのには3人称を用いる。完了した観察，実験，手術処置や特定の結論には過去時制がよく，総括したり，また一般に妥当な記述には現在時制を用いるのが正しい。受動態を過度に使用するのはおかしい。'the membrane is crossed by the protein' は 'the protein crosses the membrane' とすればわかりやすい。'as is shown by Fig.1' としないで，'Fig.1 shows' と書く。著者の考え方を述べるときは 'it is thought' とせず 'I (we) believe' としよう。受動態は医書の文中でふさわしいことも多いが，リズムを変化させるために用いるのでなければ，できるだけ能動態にするべきである。

3.5　明快で正確に

Good expository prose depends on clarity and precision. Since your purpose in writing is to communicate—to describe, explain, or interpret—clarity is essential.

Anitra Peebles Sheen, Medical writer[2]

　文章を最も効果的にするには，明快で正確に書くことである。冗長な書き方と気取った表現はやめよう。確信のもてない言い回しや推測めいた記述で逃げ道を作るのはよくない。'It may seem reasonable to suggest that necrotic effects may possibly be due to in-

volvement of some toxin-like substances' この文には不確定語が8つ
も含まれており，'Necrosis may be due to toxins（壊死は毒素のため
であろう）'を意味するに過ぎない。

3.6 動　詞

　動詞の使い方で文章は生き生きとし活力が出る。語形が長く重い
感じがする動詞は，文章の流れを妨げないようであれば，短かくて
active な動詞を使用するようにしよう。

例　示

anticipate	⟶	expect
assist	⟶	help，aid
commence	⟶	begin，start
demonstrate	⟶	show
endeavor	⟶	try（hard）
exhibit	⟶	show
initiate	⟶	begin
furnish	⟶	give，supply
require	⟶	need
terminate	⟶	end
utilize	⟶	use

（付録2「語句の使用法」参照）

第 3 章　執筆の要点と問題点

3.7　慣用句

　慣用句 phrase は日常会話や手紙などで頻繁に使用されているが，sentence が長くなったり正確性を欠くことがあるので，できるだけ平易な語に代えて書くようにしたい。出版社の編集者により訂正されることが多い。

例　示

as already stated	$\longrightarrow$	省略せよ
at some future time	$\longrightarrow$	later
at the present moment, at this time	$\longrightarrow$	now
considerable amount of	$\longrightarrow$	much
due to the fact that	$\longrightarrow$	because
in all cases	$\longrightarrow$	always
in connection with	$\longrightarrow$	about，for
in order to	$\longrightarrow$	to
in view of the fact that	$\longrightarrow$	since，because
it is of interest to note that	$\longrightarrow$	省略せよ
large number(s) of	$\longrightarrow$	many
pertaining to	$\longrightarrow$	on，about
pr or to	$\longrightarrow$	before
small number(s) of	$\longrightarrow$	few
subsequent to	$\longrightarrow$	after

（付録 2「語句の使用法」参照）

15

3.8　副　詞

　文章中で副詞を多用していることに気付くことがある。comparatively, exactly, fairly, quite, rather, really, relatively, very など
の副詞は本当に必要かどうか，不用またはどちらでもよいと判断す
れば思い切って削除した方がよい。

3.9　接続詞

　連結語の使用は避けて通れない。接続詞の and は等位接続詞で
あり，文法上同じ性質の語・句・節を対等につなぐのが原則であ
る。but は等位または従位接続詞で否定的構文のあとで使うことが
多い。however, nevertheless, therefore, thus などの接続副詞は
読者を論理的に導くために使う。文頭に basically と書くと cliché
（きまり文句）とされ，その後の文が陳腐な表現（考え）という印象を
もたれる。

> As a scientific author, you must write so that you are under-
> stood or, perhaps more important, so that you are not misun-
> derstood.
>
> Anitra Peebles Sheen, Medical writer[2]

3.10　代名詞

　代名詞の it, this, that や which は前置詞または先行詞が明白で
ないとならない。読者が首を傾げたり誤解する恐れがあるよりは，

第3章　執筆の要点と問題点

名詞を繰り返して使用する方がずっとよい。

3.11　現在分詞と不定詞

3人称で書いている場合は，現在分詞 present participle の使用は注意を要する。日本人がよく間違う例をあげる。

Examining the results, the conclusions are obvious. この文の主語は the conclusions なので，文法的には the conclusions are examining the results を意味する。分詞句の examining the results が主語と結合されていないために生じた間違いである。この誤りは主語を示して次のように訂正する。When we examined the results, the conclusions were obvious.

不定詞 infinitive も同様に注意を要する。

To apply this form of treatment, the patient had to be admitted to hospital. この文の the patient は apply の主語ではないので間違いである。本当の主語を使って訂正する。To apply this form of treatment, we had to admit the patient to hospital.

3.12　批判と引用

他人が書いた本の内容や記述を批判する必要があるときは，医学的あるいは科学的根拠を批判し，個人攻撃をしてはいけない。他人の研究内容や説明文を引用するときは正確を期すべきである。特に記述の1部分を引用する場合は，原文の真意を損なわないように注意しなければならない。

17

3.13 著作権の取り扱い方

　著作権法上，他人の原文からどの程度なら無断で引用してもよいかとなると，必ずしも明確ではない。数行にわたり，つまり約200語以上引用する場合には，許可を求めておく方が無難である。図または表をそっくり複写したいのであれば，通常は版権所有者から許可を入手しなければならない。著者が版権所有者でない場合は，法で要求されていなくとも，版権所有者の承認はもとより，著者の承諾をも得ることが一般の礼儀である。執筆中の初期の段階で許可申請をしておきたい。このような許可を得るのは，出版社や編集者の仕事ではなく，あくまでも著者の責務である（付録1「許可申請の手紙」参照）。

3.14 用語の調べ方

　重要単語は最初に和英辞典で調べ，次に捜し出した複数の英単語を英英辞典で照合し，最後にそこで選んだ英単語を英和辞典で確認すると万全である。手間がかかる作業だが，最新の辞典や増補・改訂された辞典には，医学・生命科学分野での進歩や現状に関連する用語が収録されている。

▶著作に役立つ英語大辞典（英英）

　Webster's Third New International Dictionary of the English Language, 1961, Merriam-Webster, Springfield, Mass.
　　増補版：1971，76，81，86，93，2002　Fourth ed: in prep.（2018年4月現在）
　The Shorter Oxford English Dictionary, 6th edition, 2007, Oxford University Press, London

第3章　執筆の要点と問題点

英国の出版社が，つづり字の典拠にしている。

The Random House Dictionary of the English Language, 2nd edition, 1987, Random House, Inc., New York

科学的な著述にも役立つ。英国式のつづりも示されている。

日本語版：小学館，東京

Dorland's Illustrated Medical Dictionary, 32nd edition, 2011, W. B. Saunders Company, Philadelphia

日本語版：廣川書店，東京

Stedman's Medical Dictionary, 28th edition, 2005, Lippincott Williams & Wilkins, Philadelphia

日本語版：メジカルビュー社，東京

医師が100歳の壁を越えるには

- ▶病院の待合室で読んだ某週刊誌の特集「現役医師の健康法」を，記憶の範囲で列記する。
- ▶適度なアルコール摂取，野菜，果物，魚，納豆，卵，ヨーグルトを大目に/コンビニ弁当，ペットボトルのお茶や缶コーヒーを買わない/毎朝15分の体操，背腹筋力トレと股関節のストレッチ/週2回ジョギングと筋トレ/6時間超の睡眠，寝る前に仕事のことは考えない/柔らかい歯ブラシで舌や粘膜をマッサージ/靴底の減り方が均等になるように歩く，etc．
- ▶東京都健康長寿医療センター研究所が8年かけて追跡し，発表した調査結果によると「BMI，総コレステロール，血清アルブミン，血中ヘモグロビンの各数値が低いほど生存率が低下する。低栄養が死亡のリスクを高める」。健康であることがよい医師の条件。自分に合った健康法で100歳の壁を突破しよう。

19

第4章

出版社を選ぶ

医学・生命科学の諸分野を広範にカバーしている出版社から，特定の主題だけに絞っている出版社，また主として学会の議事録を扱う出版社など，多数の出版社が存在する（付録3「海外の医学・生命科学系出版社リスト」参照）。

　目標出版社 target publisher を選ぶにはどうすればよいか，以下にそのチェックポイントを述べてみよう。

4.1 図書館と書店を活用する

　自分の専門分野で，テキストブック，アトラス，研究書などのそれぞれについて，定本はどの社から出版されているか，改版は定期的に行われているかをチェックする。次に，グッド・アイデアの良書を意欲的に，またタイムリーに出している出版社を数社探してノートする。新刊書を手にとり触れ合う機会をできるだけ多くしよう。Seeing is believing。

4.2 研究仲間や同僚に訊く

　英語が母国語の研究仲間や友人に執筆意図を伝え意見や助言を求める。出版の経験があれば，出版社名，書名，発行年などを前もって調べ，①当該出版社を選択した理由，②編集担当者とのコミュニケーションは良好だったか，③出版後の宣伝や販売に関する満足度，などを訊いて参考にする。

第4章　出版社を選ぶ

4.3 学会展示場で出版社に接触する

　海外で開催される学会の annual meeting では，多数の出版社が本を展示する。各出版社は，自社の関連商品を宣伝するだけでなく，同時に prospective authors の開発に携わる。このような学会に出席したら，書籍展示場に出向き，いくつかの出版社の編集部代表者 editorial representatives と面談するよう勧める。執筆の意図を具体的に述べて，各出版社に関心の有無を打診してみよう。この場合，全面的な関心が得られなくても悲観することはなく，むしろ話し合いから得られた示唆やヒントを，次章で検討する企画書の中で生かす心構えが大切である。内容を部分的に変更することにより，出版社の方針や要望に合致する企画となり，契約に至るケースが実際には多いのである。

　次の手紙は，Lea & Febiger の R. Kenneth Bussy 氏が，日本人 prospective author 某教授の企画について報告を受け，学会終了後にフォロー・アップのため出したものである。

Dear Dr. ＿＿＿＿＿＿＿＿＿ :

　Mr. Mark Ohgaki, who works for Lea & Febiger in Japan, tells me that you are planning to write a book on Ultrastructure of Normal and Abnormal Skin—a book that would be better than the one we publish by Zelickson. If your book is to be simply an atlas of ultrastructure, I must regretfully express our lack of interest. The Zelickson book was a very poor seller and we hardly ever have anyone ask us for books

---

23

on ultrastructure of the skin. If, however, you have something else in mind—perhaps a mixture of line and ultrastructure pictures—we would be interested. May I suggest that you correspond with me giving me more information about what you have in mind. While I do not know you personally, I have heard many good things about you and would be interested in discussing your plans further.

Sincerely,

R. Kenneth Bussy

Executive Editor

Lea & Febiger

第5章

企画書の作成と審査

目標出版社を数社に絞ったら，次はいよいよ企画書を作成することになる。出版社は，prospective author から提出された英文企画書の内容を検討して出版の可否を決めるので，明瞭で説得力がある構成にしたい。医学・生命科学系出版社に提出する企画書は，概ね次の内容を備えることが望ましい。

NEW BOOK PROPOSAL

1. 著者/編集者名と肩書
   eメールアドレス，電話番号などの連絡先
   Names, titles, e-mail addresses, and telephone numbers of authors/editors

2. 書名(暫定的なものでよい)
   Tentative book title

3. 原稿の段階　*Present stage of manuscript:*
   idea（　　）, 50%（　　）, more than 50%（　　）
   原稿完成の時期：＿＿＿＿＿＿＿
   Probable date for manuscript completion

4. 原稿の規模　*Mechanical dimensions of manuscript*
   予想ページ数：＿＿＿＿＿＿　Estimate of printed pages
   A4 または 8½×11 インチ(215×280 mm)の用紙にダブル・スペースで打って，2枚が1ページの計算でよい。
   tables：＿＿＿＿＿＿(数)
   line drawings：＿＿＿＿＿＿
   halftones (photos)：＿＿＿＿＿＿

第5章 企画書の作成と審査

cclor illustrations： _____

5. 希望（予想）価格　*Estimate of approximate price range for the book*

読者層を踏まえて大体の希望額を示す。

例えば　US＄35.00〜＄40.00

6. 企画の「狙い」，「目的」と「範囲」

Aim, Purpose and Scope of the book

7. 読者層・マーケット　*Listing of professional and/or student markets*

primary market： _____

secondary market： _____

8. 競合書　*Comparison of proposed book to competing titles*

著者名，書名，版数，出版社，発行年，ページ数，価格を示す。

9. 添付資料

序　文　Preface

目　次　Table of Contents

見本章　Sample chapter(s)

　独創的な企画でなければ，競合書を圧倒して読者にアピールすることはできない。著者には深い学識と読者に対する新鮮かつ鋭敏な感覚が求められる。上述の企画書の内容で最も重要なのが，6，7，8 の立案なので，例文を示しながら検討してみよう。

5.1 企画の「狙い」,「目的」と「範囲」

Solid evidence of planning and intent is necessary to write a book and to get a publisher to accept your proposal.

Karen Berger, Editor[1]

　Aim と Purpose は厳密に区別する必要はない。何をどう書くのか,つまり,どのような内容の本を企画し,誰に読んでもらうのか,企画の意図 intent を明確にしよう。

　以下に示す英語の「例文 1〜7」は,英語が自国語の prospective authors が Lea & Febiger, Philadelphia に提出した企画書から選んだもので,氏名を伏せ見本として使用する許可を得たものである。いずれも要点がピンポイントされ,著者の意図が明確に伝わる内容になっている。

第 5 章　企画書の作成と審査

📖 例　文　1

　最初は「基礎免疫学」に関する本で，約 300 ページ，主たる読者対象は医学生。テキスト採用を狙っており，著者は 2 名，いわゆる Co-authored textbook である。

> This book presents a comprehensive summary of modern basic immunology with an emphasis on the cellular basis of the immune response. The chapters are well integrated and present a continuum of knowledge that is basic to understanding the fundamental principles of immunology.
>
> Concise and up-to-date coverage is given to the structure and function of the immune system, cellular basis of the immune response, immunopathology, immunohematology, autoimmunity, immunity to bacteria, fungi, viruses and animal parasites as well as tumor immunology.
>
> This textbook is primarily designed for students of medicine who are taking their first formal course in immunology. It is also well designed for a self-instruction update in immunology for medical housestaff, interns and medical practitioners.

29

例 文 2

　次は「病理学総論」に関する本で，著者は4名。約500ページ，
360枚前後のイラストがあり，医科・歯科大学でのテキストを目指
す。2色刷を希望。Multi-authored textbook。

　　We have approached recent advances in the field of general
pathology by considering five major areas: cellular injury, tissue
injury (inflammation), agents of disease, neoplasia, and aging. A
final chapter with six sections is included for those desiring a
more extensive discussion of cellular injury and response. We
have integrated the basic principles of immunology and hemo-
stasis with the inflammatory process and have discussed agents
of disease both generally and in relation to specific diseases. By
evaluating clinical prototypes of injurious agents such as sickle
cell disease (genetic), myocardial infarction (physical), celiac disease (nutritional), viral hepatitis (infectious), alcohol toxicity (drug),
and myasthenia gravis (immune) from the molecular level through
ultrastructure and histopathology to clinical presentation, we
have aimed at presenting a unified approach to the multiple fac-
tors involved in the pathogenesis of disease.

　　The illustrations, figures, and tables are integral parts of the
book. They are designed to clarify and supplement the text as
well as to provide a unifying perspective of disease.

第5章　企画書の作成と審査

例　文 *3*

　今度は，ある高名な外科学教授が企画した「標準外科手術法」に関するアトラスで，約250ページ，270枚前後のペン書きイラストと説明文が系統的に配列されている。外科系レジデントのトレーニングに最適。Single-authored Atlas。

This particular ATLAS is a new book and is designed to cover in detail the various operative procedures which a general surgeon in residency training would be likely to encounter. Thus it also applies to any graduate of a surgical residency program who covers the same breadth of work which is encountered in a tertiary care hospital on a general surgical service. By definition, the book spans a number of different subspecialties of general surgery including vascular, transplantation, oncologic as well as endocrine, gastrointestinal, colorectal, pancreaticobiliary, hapatic, etc.

The special features of the book which are likely to appeal to prospective customers are the breadth of the material covered and the relatively concise format which permits any general surgeon to refer easily and quickly to one of the procedures which he is about to undertake.

The book has text application primarily to residents in general surgical training but it should also be useful for medical students in their surgical clerkships and for any general surgeon who

31

would like a rapid review of technical approaches to a problem he is about to undertake.

第5章　企画書の作成と審査

例 文 4

　この例は，「小児の複雑な足奇形」を主題とする Reference book
で単独執筆。全体を 400 ページ位で構成し，700 枚のイラストを駆
使して奇形の病因と外科療法を詳述。読者対象は整形外科医と整形
外科のレジデント。

　　This book is intended to provide a thorough discussion of the
foot problems in children that frequently or nearly always require
some type of surgical consideration.　Most of these deformities
are invariably progressive in their behavior, and surgical treatment
is often the only means of solving the problem.　The simpler and
more common foot problems in childern are discussed very
briefly, simply because most of them are often self-correcting and
rarely cause problems in adult life.　No effort is made to cover
postural or static abnormalities, and therefore disorders such as
bunions, hammer toes, and other congenital or infantile postural
abnormalities are not discussed.　Likewise, no effort is made to
include treatment of the unusual and oftentimes bizarre deformities encountered in terminal limb deficiencies.

　　The principle thrust of this text is in the direction of thoughtful
analysis of the problem, discussion of the historical evolution of
treatment, and a rational development of the therapeutic modalities.　In this regard, it will have its primary attraction to orthopedic
surgeons and orthopedic residents who are interested in treating

33

these kinds of foot deformities.

It is difficult to find an in-depth treatise that covers the pathogenetic and surgical modalities available for treatment of these kinds of complicated and fascinating foot problems. Most currently available texts do not provide a comprehensive approach to these conditions, and it is the intent of this text to fulfill that need.

第5章　企画書の作成と審査

例　文　5

　この本は，「不整脈」に関する知識を系統的に学べるよう，また教えられるように工夫したもので，CCU のナースから心臓病の専門医までかなり広い読者を対象にしている。著者は 2 名，250 ページ，240 ECGs で構成されている。Co-authored teaching book。

The publication of still another book on cardiac arrhythmias is hardly worth writing about.

But this isn't just "another book on cardiac arrhythmias." It is a superb teaching book, meticulously illustrated and written to provide medical personnel ranging from CCU nurses to practicing cardiologists an opportunity to become proficient, or more proficient as the case may be, in the interpretation of cardiac arrhythmias.

The book contains four sections, each encompassing major groups of arrhythmias. Each section begins with a text which discusses the various arrhythmias, with emphasis on electrocardiographic characteristics and variations, differentiation from other arrhythmias, and the methods of analysis and their pitfalls. Electrophysiologic and clinical background is provided when appropriate. The ECGs then follow. Their order of appearance roughly parallels the discussion in the text; in addition, within each group of arrhythmias, the ECGs progress from the simple to the more complex. Individuals who are more advanced may

35

quickly review the early, straight-forward ECGs and text their wits on those presenting more complexity. The authors' interpretations provide a step-by-step analysis, so that the reader may learn how the conclusion was reached. The book seeks not only to present a compendium of arrhythmias, but to teach an analytic approach to interpretation which can be incorporated in the thought processes of the reader.

For the neophyte or the less sophisticated reader, this book will prove a valuable learning experience. The practicing cardiologist will find it to be a useful reference, and a help in teaching others.

第5章　企画書の作成と審査

例 文 6

　この例は，「頻拍」に関するシンポジウムで発表された論文を2名の専門家が編集し，頻拍の機序に基づく診断と治療法を約500ページにまとめたもの。読者対象は心血管，心臓病専門医と頻拍に関心をもつ内科医。Co-edited work。

> The main purpose and scope of this book can be briefly defined as the aim would be to lead to a better understanding of: 1) mechanisms of tachyarrhythmias, 2) the role of intracardiac stimulation and mapping studies for evaluating tachycardias, 3) newer concepts in the pharmacologic pacing and surgical therapy of tachyarrhythmias, 4) the pharmacology of some new antiarrhythmic agents, and 5) methods of predicting patients at risk for sudden death.
>
> The book is useful for cardiovascular fellows and cardiologists. Some internal medicine specialists may be interested in the book.

例 文 7

　最後は，「関節液分析」に関する実用的なハンドブックを狙いとする約 350 ページの Single-authored book。多数の文献に散在するデータや情報を整理し，カラー写真やダイヤグラムを駆使してわかりやすく解説。関節リウマチの専門医と検査技師を主たる読者対象とする。

> To provide a practical, easy to handle reference for the study of joint fluid and its clinical application. There is currently no single source from which interested laboratory personnel, medical students, clinicians, or pathologists can obtain the details necessary to establish the process of joint fluid analysis and to interpret the results.
>
> Although this text is a practical handbook for laboratory use, it discusses the clinical aspects of the rheumatic and arthritic disorders, and the interpretation of the joint fluid findings pertinent in the practice of medicine and therefore is important reading even for physicians and medical students who are not directly involved with laboratory testing.

第 5 章　企画書の作成と審査

5.2　読者層・マーケット

　Aim, Purpose and Scope で読者対象を述べた場合は，これらを 1 次と 2 次マーケットに分けて示すと，検討する編集者にわかりやすい。

Primary and Secondary Markets

The primary market is medical students and pediatric cardiologists.

The secondary market is adult cardiologists, pediatricians, intensive care nurses, and electrocardiographic technicians.

Primary and Secondary Markets

The primary market is physicians in nuclear medicine and medical students in nuclear medicine.

The secondary market is nuclear technicians.

Primary and Secondary Markets

The primary market is ophthalmologists and ophthalmology residents.

The secondary market is pediatric neurologists.

5.3　競合書

　最初に競合書の著者名，書名，版数，出版社，発行年と，できれ ばページ数と価格を示す。多数あれば 5 点程度に絞って記入する。

次に競合書と比較して，提案する本はどこが違うのか，または，どんな長所があるのかについてわかりやすく述べる。直接的に競合する本がなければ，'There is no direct competition for this book'と書けばよいが，こんな場合でも，間接的にはcompeteすると思われる類書に対し，どんな長所または利点をもつかを明確にしよう。

　次の例は，放射線科の医師とレジデント向けに，約200ページの図譜'ATLAS OF HUMAN CROSS-SECTIONAL ANATOMY'を企画し，最も競合する図譜と比較した場合の利点を箇条書にしたもの。とてもわかりやすくて参考になる。

Competition

While there are a number of cross-sectional anatomy atlases available, their primary emphasis is either on computed tomography, ecography or nuclear magnetic resonance scanning of the anatomy rather than on the structural relationships of the anatomy itself.　There are also several atlases on individual regions of the body, most notably the head and neck, but coverage is limited.　These publications could only be considered indirectly competitive.

The closest direct competitor is Peterson's A CROSS-SECTIONAL APPROACH TO ANATOMY, published by Year Book in 2008 [110 pgs. with 300 illustrations] that is intended as a self study work book.

In the precise sense there is, as yet, no direct competition for this atlas.

第5章　企画書の作成と審査

Advantages of This Title

1. Shows anatomic structure from superior and inferior [cranial & caudal] views.
2. Shows structure within each cross-section as well as the surface features.
3. Shows both male and female pelvic structure.
4. Shows head and neck sectioned at 0° and 20° from orbital metal plane.
5. Emphasizes major features and radiologic landmarks as well as many more details than appear in the various CT, NMR and ultrasonographic scans of the human body.

5.4　企画書の送付先

　企画書を仕上げたら目標出版社へカバリング・レターをつけて送付しよう。企画書の内容を検討するのは，通常 Acquisition Editor と呼ばれる経験豊富な編集者であるが，出版社により次のような役職名を使用している。

　　Associate Editor
　　Director of Acquisition
　　Editorial Director
　　Executive Editor
　　Senior Editor

大手出版社では，subject area 別に職務を分担しているので，自

41

分の企画書を検討してもらう Acquisition Editor 名を予め調べてお
く必要がある。Dear Sir〔Madam〕とか Gentlemen で始まるカバリ
ング・レターは，担当 editor に企画書を売り込む側の準備不足を
さらけだすことになる。正確な個人・役職名を表示すべきである。
更に個人名がないと，時折，企画書は複数の編集者たちのデスクを
経て，本来なら担当となる editor からの返事が遅れる原因となる。

5.5 企画の審査

企画書は acquisition editor により次の諸点で審査を受ける。

- 企画の内容が自社の出版方針に合致しているかどうか。
- 着想 idea に新味または独創性があり，しかもタイムリーか。
- 文章のスタイル，記述の仕方は明快で正確か。
- 読者層，1次と2次マーケットのサイズ，競合書や類書との
  比較。
- 提案された判型，体裁，ページ数，イラスト数から制作原
  価を予測。
- 予定価格で target readers を十分に取り込めるか。
- 著者や寄稿者の評判は良好か。

著者が送付した企画書のアウトラインと sample chapter(s) は，
通常 expert reviews のため著者と同分野の専門家に送付され，意見
と評価が求められる。

出版社の acquisition editor から返事が届くのは，proposal 送付後
4〜6週間経ってからである。春と秋は，出版社の編集者は，いろ

第 5 章　企画書の作成と審査

いろな学会や同業者との会合に出席する多忙な時期なので，更に2～3週間の日数を余計にみておいた方がよい。

　企画が何らの質疑も受けずに受理されることは滅多にない。最も多く受け取る回答は，出版決定に先立ち，「特定の変更または修正が可能かどうか」を問い合わせてくるものである。このようなオファーは慎重に検討し，内容の改良に役立つのであれば積極的に受け入れるべきである。変更内容が企画の大部分に及ぶとか，着想そのものを否定している場合は，他社へ当たるべきであろう。「企画が特殊過ぎる」とか，逆に「一般的過ぎる」とかという理由で受理できないと述べている場合は，議論をしても無駄で，やはり別の出版社と交渉すべきである。

　企画に興味はあるが，「sample chapters の英語が不完全 incomplete」と指摘されることもある。最終原稿をネイティブのスペシャリストにチェックしてもらい，英語の誤りを訂正または文章を補強することを条件に出版決定となるケースもある。

　企画が受理されなかったり，受理されてもかなりの内容変更条件付きの場合に，出版社に辛辣なレターを出すことは好ましくない。acquisition editor は出版方針に沿って企画書を真剣に審査している。勧告された内容，評価やアドバイスは，できるだけ活用する姿勢が大切である。

43

広辞苑,「LGBT」の説明に誤り

▶「LGBT」は,女性同性愛者 Lesbian,男性同性愛者 Gay,両性愛者 Bisexual,生まれた時の性別とは異なる生き方をする Trans-gender の頭文字をとった略語。10年ぶりに刊行された第7版には,「多数派とは異なる性的指向をもつ人々」と記された。

▶「LGB」は好きになる性を表わす「性的指向」の概念だが,「T」は自分は男か女かといった自己認識を表わす「性自認」の概念。広辞苑の説明だと「LGB」の説明にしかなっていないとの指摘がインターネット上であった。

▶ "To err is human, to forgive divine/あやまちは人の常,許すは神の業(わざ)"。英国の詩人 Alexander Pope(1688-1744)の言葉。辞典の編集は並大抵の仕事ではない。だが,誤りは修正しなければならない。「重圧で夜も眠れなかった」と責任者は語る。出版に携わった者として,辞典編集部諸氏の労を多としたい。

第**6**章

契約締結→そして出版へ

6.1 契約書

契約書は publishing agreement または contract と呼ばれ，著作者と出版社間で必ず締結される重要な書類である。次のような諸項目，条件や約束事が記載される。

1. 本文，図表，写真などを含む完全原稿 complete or finished manuscript またはデジタルデータの引き渡し日。

2. 書名 title，判型 format，構成 organization，初刷 initial printing，増刷 additional printing などに関する事項。

3. 印税 royalty についての取り決め。royalty rate は出版社により異なるが，通常は出版価格の 10％である。販売部数により sliding royalty scale を設定している出版社もある。時には，入金額の 15％を提示されることがあるが，出版社は取次業者や書店に割引販売するので，出版価格の 10％の方が有利である。発行部数の少ない本や議事録などでは，原稿一括買切り方式もある。

4. 著作者への金銭支援として前払金 advance が支給される場合の条件。

5. 本の予定発行日，予定価格，出版社による宣伝や販売計画の概略。

6. 契約の有効期間，自動継続，内容変更，解除などに関する事項。

7. 著作者と出版社の役割と責務。

契約書を受け取ったら内容を熟読し，疑念や質問があれば，署名

第6章 契約締結→そして出版へ

の前に，acquisition editor に説明を求めることが大切である。

6.2 著者の責務 obligations

1. 原稿を準備する。A4 または $8\frac{1}{2}\times11$ インチ(215×280 mm)の用紙に typewritten, double-spaced with one-inch margins が原則。図，表，その他のイラスト数は同意されたリミット内で作成。特にカラー図版は勝手に入れたり増やしてはならない。artist's cost は著者の負担であるが，一部を出版社がもつこともある。索引 index の作成費用は通常著者負担である。

2. 完全原稿の締切日は出版社により，また本の内容により異なるが，6 か月から 2 年以内が多い。acquisition editor と相談して決めるが，契約書に記載されたら厳守しなければならない。遅れると編集，制作，販売スケジュールなどの変更原因となり，出版社スタッフとの関係が悪化する。

3. ゲラ galley や校正刷り page proof を受け取ったらチェックし，できるだけ早く返送する。proofreading の期日を指定されたら守ることが，その後の進行をスムースにする。

4. 校正の段階で大幅に変更をしてはならない。通常 10%を超える変更をすると，typesetting などの変更に要する費用を負担しなければならない。

5. 著作権で保護された材料の複製には，著者の費用で credit line が明記され，署名された許可書を入手し出版社に提出する。日本では，出版社の仕事と誤解している人がいるが，著者の責務なので，執筆中に許可申請をするようにしたい(付録1「許可申請の手紙(見本)」参照)。

47

6.3 編集と制作

1. 出版社では仕上り原稿を編集作業の前に，processors と呼ばれる人達が点検する。本文，本文内容に合致するイラスト，図表と説明文，複製材料の許可書と credit lines などの全部が揃っているかがチェックされる。編集作業は社内スタッフの manuscript editors か，出版社によってはフリーランスの editors が担当する。原稿の構成，論理的な展開，表現の明瞭性，またスペリングや文法上の誤りと弱点が訂正されたり補強されたりする。編集中に生じる大きな問題点については，acquisition editor が著者に直接意見を求めてくるが，小さな疑問は校正刷りに記入される。著者は指摘された訂正，補強個所を検討し，疑問点に応答しなければならない。

2. 著者が制作部 Production Department へ直接コンタクトすることは滅多にないが，本の出来映えと完成度に貢献する重要な部署である。印刷やイラストの体裁，活字の書体と大きさからカバーデザインまでがエキスパートの手により決定される。こうして本は，組み版，写真製版，印刷，製本などの工程を経て完成する。

完成本 finished book を手にしたときの著者のよろこびは何物にも代え難い。費やした時間と努力が'かたち'になって実現し，世界中の読者の手にわたることになる。おめでとう！　まずは，仕事を理解し長い間協力してくれた家族と共に乾杯しましょう。

付　録

付録 1　許可申請の手紙（見本）

Dear . . . . . .

I am writing a book entitled"Bedside Diagnosis: Cardiology"for publication in the United States. I should be grateful if you would grant permission for the following to be reproduced:

Table 10, Chap. 6 from your book"Guide to Physical Examination and History Taking, 9th Edition", 2007 by Lippincott Williams & Wilkins, Philadelphia.

I am also writing separately to the publisher requesting permission to reproduce this material. The usual acknowledgements and a full reference to the table will of course be included. If you would like the credit line to take any special form, please let me know what this should be.

Would you please indicate your agreement by signing and returning one copy of this letter?

Thank you for your cooperation.

Sincerely yours,
Taro Yamamoto, MD

I/ We grant permission to reproduce the material specified above.

Signed: . . . .
(copyright-holder/ author)
Date: . . . .

Credit line to be used:

付　録

付録2　語句の使用法

　医学・生命科学分野で論文，専門書，教科書などを執筆するときに，日本人著者が不注意で多用しがちな「避けたい語句」を左欄に，そして対応する「好ましい語句」を右欄にアルファベット順に記載した。ただし必ずしも的確な同義語とは限らないので，あくまでも参考にしていただきたい[3]。

避けたい語句	好ましい語句
anticipate　あることを喜びまたは苦痛をもって予測する	expect　かなりの確信をもって待ち望む
approximately　語形が長い	about
are of the same opinion　短くせよ	agree　最も普通な語
area	後出の 'woolly words' の項を見よ
arrive at a decision　回りくどい	decide　動詞だと1語でよい
as already stated	〔省略せよ〕
as can be seen from Fig.1, growth is more rapid	growth is more rapid (Fig.1), あるいは Fig.1 shows that growth is more rapid
as far as our own observations are concerned, they show	our/ my observations show
as follows: —	ダッシュは省略せよ，コロンで十分
as for these experiments, they are	these experiments are
as of now	now, from now on
as regards this species, it	this species is
as shown in Fig.11	Fig.11 shows that
assist (-ance)	help, aid
at a later date, at some future time	later
at the present moment, at the present moment in time, at this time	now

51

避けたい語句	好ましい語句
author(s), the	I/ we
bright red in color	bright red
carry out experiments 　回りくどい	experiment 　動詞にすると1語ですむ
case	patient
conduct an investigation 　回りくどい	investigate 　1語ですむ
commence 　形式ばった語で，儀式などを始めるときに使う	begin, start 　一般的な語で，動作の開始・着手に使う
comparatively	〔他と実際に比較するとき以外は使用するな〕
concerning this effect, it may be borne in mind that 　気取った表現はやめる	〔省略せよ〕
considerable amount of	much
considerable number/ proportion of	many, most
data	facts, results, observations
decreased number of	fewer, less
demonstrate 　(広げて大規模に)見せる	show 　一般的な語
due to the fact that 　回りくどい	because 　接続詞を使うと1語ですむ
during the month of January 　不必要に長い	in January 　単純に書く
elevated 　(相対的に)高くした，高い	raised, higher 　正確な語を使う
employ 　(金を払って人を)使用する	use 　(ある目的のために物・ときに人を)用いる
encountered 　(思いがけなく)出会った	met 　短い語にする
encountered frequently (e.g. 'this effect was encountered frequently') 　回りくどい	common ('this effect was common')

付　録

避けたい語句	好ましい語句
equally as well as があると意味が重複する	equally well
exhibit; X exhibits good stretch properties exhibit に人目につくように見せる，示す	show; X stretches well show は最も一般的な語
fewer in number in number は不要	fewer この比較級はもともと数に用いる
following (the operation) 意味があいまい	after (the operation) 術後，after にするとはっきりする
for a further period of ten years 不必要に長い	for another ten years 短くする
for the reason that 形式ばった表現法	because, since 一般的な語にする
from the standpoint of 形式ばった表現法	according to 一般的な語にする
goes under the name of 形式ばった表現法	is called 一般的な語にする
greater/ higher number of 短く平易にする	more 一般的な比較級の方がよい
hospitalize 入院させる	admit to hospital 許す・認めるという意味をもつ
if conditions are such that/ if it is assumed that	if
in all cases	always
in connection with	about, for
in few cases	sometimes, rarely
in excess of	more than, above
in order to	to
in regard to	〔適当な前置詞，例えば in, for, about, with を用いる〕
in relation to	
in respect of	
in terms of	
in the case of	
in the context of	

53

避けたい語句	好ましい語句
in the event that （万一）…という場合には（形式ばった表現）	if
in this connection the statement may be made that 長い前置きは不要，倦怠感を覚える	〔省略する〕
in view of the fact that 回りくどい，短い語にする	since, because …なので，…だから
it has long been known that この表現は長いだけで不正確	〔省略する〕
it is apparent, therefore, that 回りくどい，短い語を使う	hence, therefore それゆえに，したがって
it is of interest to note that 長い前置きの句は不要	〔省略する〕
it is often the case that 回りくどい	often 1語ですむ
it is possible (probable) that 回りくどい	possibly (probably)
it is this that 回りくどい	this 1語ですむ
it may, however, be noted that 長くて回りくどい（受動態にする必要がない）	nevertheless, but 短い明確な語で十分
it may be said that 回りくどい（受動態にする必要がない）	possibly 短い語で十分
it seems to the present writer 気取った表現はやめる	I think 短くする
it will be seen upon examination of Table 5 that 長い前置きの句は不要	Table 5 shows that この方がすっきりする
it would thus appear that あいまいな表現	apparently 1語ですむ
large number(s) of 抽象的で弱い	many 数を表わす

付　録

避けたい語句	好ましい語句
large proportion of 　抽象的で弱い	much, most 　量・数を表わす
lazy in character 　in character は不要	lazy 　怠惰な(性格)
lesser extent, degree 　2 重比較級は用いない方がよい	less 　程度・度合を表わす
level 　意味があいまい	concentration, content 　濃度，含量，具体的な語を使う
made a count 　名詞を用いると語数が多くなる	counted 　動詞だと 1 語ですむ
majority of 　対立観念として minority(少数)を意識 　している場合に用いる	most 　大部分
make an adjustment to 　回りくどい	adjust 　動詞 1 語ですむ
make an examination of 　回りくどい	examine 　1 語ですむ
mechanisms of a physiological nature 　語数が多い．nature は意味があいまい	physiological mechanisms 　短くする
mental patients 　意味がまぎらわしい	patients with mental disorders 　精神障害の患者
moment in time 　回りくどい	time 　1 語でよい
multiple 　一般的な語を用いる	several, different
number of, a 　はっきりしない成句	several, some 　a few よりは多く，many よりは少ない
of large size 　短く平易にする	large 　大きさ，寸法を表わす
on a regular basis 　短く平易にする	regularly
on the basis of 　形式ばった表現	from, by, because 　短い語ですむ

55

避けたい語句	好ましい語句
owing to the fact that 　表現が堅苦しい	because 　短い語ですむ
parameter 　非常にまぎらわしい語（誤用が多い）	index, criterion, factor, characteristic, measure, value, variable 　具体的で正確な語を使う
pertaining to 　語形が長い	on, about 　短くて一般的
prior to; prior to that time 　短い語を選ぶ	before; before that 　短くて一般的
quite 　ばく然とした副詞	〔省略する〕
rather 　ばく然とした副詞	〔省略する〕
relative to ('This letter is relative to') 　…に関して	about 　一般的な前置詞の方がよい
relatively 　相対的に，比較的に（誤用が多い）	〔特定の数量を他のものと比較するとき 以外は使用しない〕
respectively 　それぞれ，おのおの（誤用が多い）	〔'The first, second, and third prizes went to Jack, George, and Frank respectively.' のように正確に用いるのでなければ避 けよう〕
reveal 　（隠れているものを）明らかにする	show 　一般的な語を使う
sacrifice (experimental animals) 　犠牲にする（比喩的に使うことが多い）	kill 　普通の動詞を用いる
similar in every detail 　回りくどい	the same 　平易にする
small numbers of 　少数（相対的）	few 　1語ですむ
sophisticated 　抽象的な形容詞	advanced, new 　具体的な語を使う
species in which the hairs are lacking 　長く堅苦しい表現	hairless species 　単純に書く

付　録

避けたい語句	好ましい語句
square in shape, square-shaped 不必要に長い	square 正方形(の)
subsequent to あとの，続いて起こる	after 1語ですむのでは
such strength that strength は多義な語	so strong that 力，強さを表わす
sufficient number of 不必要に長い	enough 短い語ですむ
terminate 語形が長い	end 短く一般的な動詞を使う
the test in question 堅く形式ばった表現	this test 単純にする
the treatment having been performed, 長く重苦しい	after treatment 短く平易にする
there can be little doubt that this is 不必要に長く回りくどい	this is probably 短く平易にする
there is　there are 存在を示す固定化した表現	〔不必要であることが多い。例えば， 'There is much work being done on…', は，'Much work is being done on…' の ように変えよ〕
they are both alike (similar) they と both が相乗してくどい	they are alike (similar) 単純にする
throughout the whole of the experiment 相乗してくどい	throughout the experiment the whole of(全体)をとりすっきりさせる
two equal halves 重複する言い回し	halves 半分，half の複数形
until such time as 短くする	until
upon 重苦しい口調(動作を強調することが多い)	on 口語調で一般的
using まぎらわしい	〔懸垂分詞であるかどうか検討し，もし そうであれば 'by', 'with', 'by means of' を試みよ〕

57

避けたい語句	好ましい語句
utilize, utilization 　利用する，利用（語形が長い）	use 　短い一般的な語を用いる
very 　ばく然とした副詞は不要	〔省略する〕
We are in the process of making 　不必要に長い	We are making 　単純に書く
while 　…とはいえ，一方	although 　事実を述べるときに用いる接続詞
with reference to 　…に関して	about 　前置詞だと1語ですむ
with regard to 　…に関して	in, to 　前置詞だと1語ですむ
with the exception of 　形式ばった表現	except 　1語ですむ
woolly words：意味のはっきりしない語 area, character, conditions, field, level, nature, problem, process, situation	〔使用を避け，より正確な語に変えよ〕

付　録

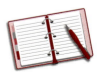

付録 3　海外の医学・生命科学系出版社リスト（国順/ABC 順）

国名	社名	所在地	主たる出版分野	URL
US	Allen Press, Inc.	810 East 10th Street, Lawrence, KS 66044	Scholarly Publishers Services	https://www2.allenpress.com/
US	American Psychiatric Publishing, Inc. (APPI)	800 Maine Avenue, S.W. Suite 900 Washington, DC 20024	Psychotherapy, PTSD, Neuropsychiatry and Biological Psychiatry	https://www.appi.org/
US	Annual Reviews Inc.	4139 El Camino Way, Palo Alto, CA 94306	Medicine, Immunology	https://www.annualreviews.org/
US	Carden Jennings Publishing Co., Ltd.	75 Greenbrier Drive, Charlottesville, VA 22901	Medical Sciences	http://www.cjp.com/
US	Cell Press	3251 Riverport Lane, Maryland Heights, MO 63043	Cell, Neuron, Cancer	http://www.cell.com/
US	The Clinics of North America	3251 Riverport Lane, Maryland Heights, MO 63043	Cardiology, Critical Care, Nursing, Surgery	http://www.theclinics.com/
US	Cold Spring Harbor Laboratory (CSHL) Press	Bungtown Road, Cold Spring Harbor, NY 11724	Viruses, Immunology, Cell Biology	https://www.cshlpress.com/
US	Heldref Publications	325 Chestnut Street, Suite 800 Philadelphia, PA 19106	Psychology, Medicine	http://www.heldref.org/
US	Lawrence Erlbaum Associates, Inc.	10 Industrial Avenue, Mahwah, NJ 07430	Medicine	http://erlbaum.com/
US	Lippincott Williams & Wilkins (LWW)	2 Commerce Square 2001 Market Street, Philadelphia, PA 19103	Medicine, Basic & Clinical, Nursing, Health	https://www.lww.com/

付　録

国名	社名	所在地	主たる出版分野	URL
US	McGraw Hill Education [Medical]	60 Taylor Station Road Blacklick, OH 43210	Allied Health, Clinical Medicine, Nursing, Pharmacy	https://www.mhprofessional.com/medical
US	Mosby-Year Book Inc.	1220 North Lindbergh Boulevard, Saint Louis, MO 6313	Medical, Health Sciences; Text Book, Year Book	https://openlibrary.org/publishers/Mosby_Year_Book
US	Physicians Postgraduate Press, Inc.	6555 Quince Rd, Memphis, TN 38119	Neurology, Psychiatry	https://sts.psychiatrist.com/Login.aspx?ReturnUrl=%2f
US	Rockefeller University Press	950 Third Ave, 2nd Floor, New York, NY 10022	Medicine	http://www.rupress.org/
US	SAGE Publications	2455 Teller Road, Thousand Oaks, CA 91320	Medicine	https://uk.sagepub.com/en-gb/eur/
US	W. B. Saunders Company	Independence Square West, Philadelphia, PA 19106	Health, Nursing, Medicine, Basic & Clinical	https://www.us.elsevierhealth.com/
US	SLACK Inc.	6900 Grove Road, Thorofare, NJ 08086	Nursing, Orthopedics	http://www.slackinc.com/
US	Springer Publishing Company, Inc.	11 West 42nd Street. 15th Floor. New York, NY 10036	Nursing	http://www.springerpub.com/
US	University of Chicago Press, Journals Division	1427 East 60th Street, Chicago, IL 60637	Life Sciences	https://www.journals.uchicago.edu/
US	Westminster Publications, Inc	P.O. Box 586 Glen Head, NY 11545	Medicine	http://www.westminsterpublications.com/
US	John Wiley & Sons, Inc.	111 River Street, Hoboken, NJ 07030	Life Science, Medicine, Food, Nursing	https://onlinelibrary.wiley.com/
US	Wiley InterScience	111 River Street, Hoboken, NJ 07030	Cell, Medical Physics	https://onlinelibrary.wiley.com/

国名	社名	所在地	主たる出版分野	URL
UK	Baywood Publishing Company, Inc.	2 Park Square, Milton Park, Abingdon-Oxford, OX14 4RN, UK	Nursing and Allied Health, Psychology, Social Sciences	https://www.routledge.com/
UK	BioMed Central	The Campus, 4 Crinan Street, London N1 9XW	Biomedicine, Chemistry, Life Sciences	https://www.biomedcentral.com/
UK	BMJ Group	BMA House, Tavistock Square, London WC1H 9JR	Emergency Medicine, Drug, Rheumatism	http://journals.bmj.com/
UK	Butterworth-Heineman	The Boulevard, Langford Lane, Kidlington, Oxford OX5 1GB	Health, Life Sciences, Physical Sciences	https://www.elsevier.com/books-and-journals/butterworth-heinemann
UK	Cambridge University Press (CUP)	Shaftesbury Rd, Cambridge CB2 8BS	Medicine, Science and Technology	http://www.cambridge.org/
UK	The Lancet	125 London Wall, London, EC2Y 5AS	Oncology, HIV, Haematology, Health, Neurology, Journals	http://www.thelancet.com/
UK	Oxford University Press (OUP)	North Kettering Business Park, Hipwell Road, Kettering, Northants NN14 1UA	Medicine	http://global.oup.com/?cc=jp
UK	Pharmaceutical Press (PhP)	66-68 East Smithfield , London E1W 1AW	Pharmaceutical	http://www.pharmpress.com/
UK	Taylor & Francis	2&4 Park Square, Milton Park, Abingdon OX14 4RN	Medicine	http://taylorandfrancis.com/
Germany	Nature Publishing Group	Heidelberger Platz 3 14197 Berlin	Biotechnology, Drug, Cancer, Neuro Science	https://www.nature.com/npg_/index_npg.html
Germany	F.K. Schattauer Verlagsgesellschaft mbH	Hölderlinstr. 3 70174 Stuttgart	Medicine	http://www.schattauer.de/nc/en/home.html
Germany	Springer	Albrechtstraße 22 10117 Berlin	Biomedicine, Neurology, Internal Medicine	http://www.springer.com/

付　録

国 名	社 名	所 在 地	主たる出版分野	URL
Germany	Springer International Publishing AG	Albrechtstraße 22 10117 Berlin	Medicine	http://www.springer.com/
Germany	Georg Thieme Verlag	Rüdigerstraße 14 70469 Stuttgart	Medicine	https://www.thieme.de/de/index.html
Germany	Thieme Medical Publishers, Inc.	Rüdigerstraße 14 70469 Stuttgart	Surgery, Orthopedics, Anatomy, Internal Medicine	https://www.thieme.com/
Netherlands	Academic Press	Radarweg 29, 1043 NX Amsterdam, The Netherlands	Health, Life Sciences, Physical Sciences	https://www.elsevier.com/books-and-journals/academic-press
Netherlands	Elsevier B.V.	Radarweg 29 Amsterdam	Life Sciences	https://www.elsevier.com/
Netherlands	Excerpta Medica	Apollo Building , Herikerbergweg 17 1101 CN Amsterdam	Cardiovascular, Diabetes, Hematology	https://www.excerptamedica.com/
Netherlands	Kluwer Academic Publishers	P.O. Box 17, 3300 AA Dordrecht	Medicine	http://vlib.ustuarchive.urfu.ru/storon/kluwer/
Netherlands	Swets & Zeitlinger Publishers	P.O. Box 825, 2160 SZ Lisse	Neurology	https://web.archive.org/web/2014 1218085019/ http://swetsinformationservices.com/
Switzerland	S. Karger AG	Allschwilerstrasse 10, CH-4055 Basel	Biomedical, Proceedings	https://www.karger.com/
Russia	Nauka-Interperiodica Publishing	117997, Moscow, ul, Profsoyuznay 90	Medicine	http://www.maik.ru/
UAE	Bentham Science Publishers Ltd.	Y-2. Building Y Saif Zone Sharjah	Drug, Life Sciences	http://bentham.org/

引用文献

1) Reeder, R.C. (ed.): Sourcebook of Medical Communication, 1981, The C. V. Mosby Company, St. Louis
   Chapter 7/ Berger, K.: Choosing and working with a book publisher
2) Sheen, A. P.: Breathing Life into Medical Writing, 1982, The C. V. Mosby Company, St. Louis
3) オコーナー，ウッドフォード/大垣訳：英語で科学論文を書く人のために，1981，廣川書店，東京
   同上復刻私家版(2014)，付録5を改訂し，本書の付録「語句の使用法」に転用。

参考文献

Barrass, R.: Scientists Must Write; A Guide to Better Writing for Scientists, Engineers and Students, 1978, Chapman and Hall Ltd, New Fetter Lane EC4P4EE

Bussy, R. K. (ed.): Philadelphia's Publishers and Printers, An Informal History, 1976, Philadelphia Book Clinic, Distributed by Rittenhouse Book Distributors, Inc., Philadelphia

Council of Biology Editors: Style Manual; A Guide for Authors, Editors, and Publishers in the Biological Sciences, 4th edn., 1978, American Institute of Biological Sciences, Arlington, VA

King, L.: Why Not Say It Clearly, 1978, Little, Brown & Co., Boston

Strunk, W., Jr, & White, E. B.: The Elements of Style, 2nd edn., 1972, Macmillan, Riverside, N. J.; Collier-Macmillan, London

あとがき

KW先生，テキスト・アトラス「Bedside Diagnosis」の英文執筆が，順調に進行しているとのお知らせに接し，よろこんでいます。私も本書の執筆が間もなく終わりますので，お約束通り，原稿のコピーをお届けいたします。今後のお仕事に役立てばよいのですが。

日本人が英語で本を書くことは，知的チャレンジとは言いながら，並大抵のことではありませんよね。どうかご健康に留意されて'Complete manuscript'に到達されますよう心から願っています。

旧知のベテラン編集者4名から，次のような集約されたコメントをいただきました。

(1) 原稿を読んで，よい企画，また内容について面白いと感じた。タイトルは「英文出版」とあるが，実は，英文書籍だけではなく，書籍全般に通じるところがある。

(2) 現在は電子メールやPDFの利用が普及している。デジタル化した内容が欠けているのは，これから出す本としてはけっこう厳しい。

時間を割き原稿をお読みいただき誠に有難う。デジタル化した内容を取り入れたマニュアル的な書籍が出ることを願っています。

第3章「著作に役立つ英語大辞典」の書誌データチェックと，付録3「海外の医学・生命科学系出版社リスト」の作成に大垣城治氏のご協力を得ました。

本書の編集と制作は，畏友藤堂保行氏が担当しました。いつもと変わらぬ心遣いと，そして丁寧なお仕事に感謝いたします。

2019年1月

大垣　雅昭

著者プロフィール

大垣　雅昭（英語名：Mark Ohgaki）

1972−91 年　フィラデルフィアの医学系出版社 Lea & Febiger と J. B. Lippincott の日本代表。

1991 年　メディカル・サイエンス・インターナショナル代表取締役社長。会長，顧問を経て 2007 年に退社。

2012 年　全出版人大会賞。英語医学用語の語源に詳しい。訳書に「オースチン，クロスフィールド：ナースの英語」，「オコーナー，ウッドフォード：英語で科学論文を書く人のために」（ともに廣川書店），著書に「はじめて学ぶ医療英語」（メディカル・サイエンス・インターナショナル）がある。

医学・生命科学書　英文出版のすすめ
　―著作を志す人へのメッセージ―　　　　　定価：本体600円＋税

2019 年 2 月 5 日発行　第 1 版第 1 刷 ©

著　者　大垣 雅昭
　　　　　おおがき　まさあき

発行者　株式会社　メディカル・サイエンス・インターナショナル

　　　　代表取締役　金子 浩平
　　　　東京都文京区本郷 1-28-36
　　　　郵便番号 113-0033　電話(03)5804-6050

印刷：双文社印刷

ISBN 978-4-8157-0150-5 C3047

本書の複製権・翻訳権・上映権・譲渡権・貸与権・公衆送信権(送信可能化権を含む)は(株)メディカル・サイエンス・インターナショナルが保有します。本書を無断で複製する行為(複写,スキャン,デジタルデータ化など)は,「私的使用のための複製」など著作権法上の限られた例外を除き禁じられています。大学,病院,診療所,企業などにおいて,業務上使用する目的(診療,研究活動を含む)で上記の行為を行うことは,その使用範囲が内部的であっても,私的使用には該当せず,違法です。また私的使用に該当する場合であっても,代行業者等の第三者に依頼して上記の行為を行うことは違法となります。

JCOPY 〈(社)出版者著作権管理機構 委託出版物〉
本書の無断複写は著作権法上での例外を除き禁じられています。複写される場合は,そのつど事前に,(社)出版者著作権管理機構(電話 03-5244-5088,FAX 03-5244-5089,info@jcopy.or.jp)の許諾を得てください。